THE CROHN'S DISEASE COOKBOOK

The Ultimate Guide to Digestive Health | 1200 Days of Digestive Empowerment with a Detailed 28-Day Meal Plan and a Food List

GINA ORRANTIA

Table Of Contents
...

CHAPTER 4 - RECIPE SECTION

Breakfasts

Lunches

Dinners

Snacks And Small Bites   45

Desserts and Treats   50

CHAPTER 5 - Managing Digestive Symptoms   55

Conclusion   59

APPENDICES: Additional Resources   61

Measurements And Conversions   64

Introduction

—————— · · ·

Living with Crohn's can feel overwhelming at times. The unpredictable flare-ups, dietary restrictions, and the constant quest for symptom relief can take a toll. But here's the good news: with the right foods and balanced nutrition, you can gain more control over your health and well-being.

This cookbook is more than just a collection of recipes; it's a comprehensive guide designed to empower you. We'll start with the basics of understanding Crohn's disease—what it is, its common symptoms, how it's treated, and most importantly, the crucial role diet plays in managing the condition. I'll share some recent research insights that can help you stay informed about new developments in the field.

Next, you'll find a deep dive into nutritional foundations specifically tailored for those with Crohn's. You'll learn about the essential nutrients your body needs, foods that can be beneficial or harmful, and how to manage potential nutritional deficiencies. I'll also share tips on staying hydrated because good hydration plays a significant role in digestive health.

One of the highlights of this book is the detailed 28-day meal plan. I've crafted daily meal breakdowns that align with nutritional goals for each week. Whether you're prepping meals for the week or adjusting your diet during flare-ups, these plans are designed to make things as simple as possible.

You'll have access to various recipes covering breakfasts, lunches, dinners, snacks, and even desserts. I've ensured that each recipe considers sensitivities commonly associated with Crohn's disease while still being delicious and satisfying.

Managing symptoms during flare-ups requires special attention, so there's an entire section dedicated to dietary adjustments when symptoms worsen. We'll talk about types of fiber—soluble vs. insoluble—and introduce you to helpful aids like probiotics and prebiotics. Plus, I'll provide some stress reduction techniques which are an often overlooked aspect of managing this condition.

Don't forget about our appendices! They include guides on supplements you might consider, tips for eating out while managing Crohn's-friendly options, and maintaining a food diary to track what works best for your body. Understanding measurements and conversions will also make following recipes easier.

With over a decade of experience as a registered dietitian specializing in gastrointestinal diseases, I've seen firsthand the impact that informed dietary choices can have on well-being. This book combines clinical expertise with real-life patient experiences and cutting-edge research.

I hope this guide becomes a valuable resource in your daily life, helping you achieve greater digestive health and empowerment over your condition. Together, let's make living with Crohn's disease a little easier and a lot more manageable.

CHAPTER 1

Understanding Crohn's Disease

Crohn's Disease is a type of inflammatory bowel disease (IBD). It's a bit like when your body's immune system gets confused and starts attacking its own digestive tract, causing inflammation. This can happen anywhere from your mouth to your anus but most commonly affects the small intestine and the beginning of the large intestine.

Think about it like this: imagine your digestive system as a long, windy road where food travels through. In someone with Crohn's, parts of that road become rough and bumpy due to inflammation, making it harder for food to pass smoothly. This inflammation can lead to areas that are swollen or even cause sores or ulcers.

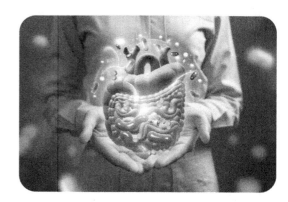

Crohn's is not caused by anything you did or didn't do. It's thought to be a mix of genetic factors (meaning it might run in your family), your environment, and an overactive immune response. Sadly, there's no cure yet, but there are ways to manage it and improve quality of life—more on that later in the book!

Common Symptoms

You might be wondering what it feels like to have Crohn's Disease. Well, the symptoms can vary from person to person, but here are some of the most common ones:

1. **Abdominal Pain:** One of the hallmark symptoms is abdominal pain. It's not just any tummy ache; people describe it as crampy or sharp pain, often located in the lower right side of the abdomen. This pain usually appears after eating and can be severe enough to wake you up at night.

2. **Diarrhea:** Frequent, watery diarrhea is another common symptom. This isn't your usual bout of diarrhea from bad food; it's persistent and can sometimes include blood or mucus.

3. **Fatigue:** Feeling extremely tired even after adequate rest can be frustrating. Chronic fatigue often accompanies Crohn's because your body is constantly battling inflammation.

4. **Weight Loss:** Unexpected weight loss happens because your body isn't absorbing nutrients effectively due to inflammation and frequent diarrhea.

5. **Fever:** Some people might experience fevers during flare-ups because their body is responding to chronic inflammation.

6. **Reduced Appetite:** With all these uncomfortable symptoms, it's no surprise that many people with Crohn's often lose their appetite or feel nauseous after eating.

7. **Mouth Sores:** Yes, inflammation isn't just limited to your digestive tract! Mouth sores or ulcers are common too.

8. **Perianal Symptoms:** Some people experience pain or drainage near their anus due to inflammation spreading to that area.

These symptoms aren't just inconvenient—they can drastically affect someone's day-to-day life and emotional well-being. Remember, having one or even several of these symptoms doesn't automatically mean you have Crohn's disease—they're just common signs doctors look for during diagnosis.

Treatment Overview

Getting treated for Crohn's is all about managing symptoms and maintaining remission so that you can live your life as normally as possible. There isn't a one-size-fits-all plan here; treatments vary from person to person based on the severity and location of their disease.

1. **Medications:** Most people with Crohn's will be very familiar with medication. The types you're likely to encounter include:

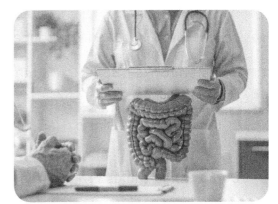

   a. *Aminosalicylates (5-ASAs):* These are usually prescribed for mild symptoms and aim to reduce inflammation at the surface level of your lining.

   b. *Corticosteroids:* If you're experiencing moderate to severe flare-ups, corticosteroids can be used short-term to control inflammation.

   c. *Immunomodulators:* These work by dampening your immune response, which can help manage your body's inflammation over the long term.

   d. *Biologics:* These are targeted therapies that block specific proteins involved in inflammation.

   e. *Antibiotics:* Sometimes prescribed if there are complications like infections or fistulas.

Each of these medications comes with its pros and cons, and it might take some trial and error with your healthcare provider to find what works best for you.

2. **Nutrition Support:** Many people with Crohn's need vitamins and minerals they might not be absorbing from food due to their condition.

   a. *Supplements:* If you're not absorbing nutrients properly due to inflammation or surgery, supplements might be critical.

   b. *Enteral Nutrition:* For some people, special liquid diets that provide all necessary nutrients might be used as part of the treatment plan.

3. **Surgery:** When medications aren't enough or if complications arise, surgery might be an option. Common surgical interventions include removing damaged sections of the intestine or repairing fistulas. It's not a cure, but it can provide significant relief.

The Role of Diet in Crohn's

Our bodies react to food continuously since it's our primary source of energy and nutrients. For someone with Crohn's, certain foods can trigger flare-ups while others could help soothe symptoms and promote healing. A friend of mine discovered through trial and error that her diet had a huge impact on her symptoms. Here are some basic guidelines I've picked up about eating with Crohn's:

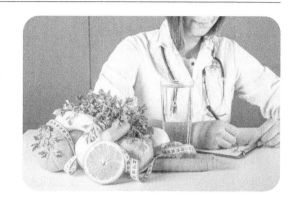

1. **Listen to Your Body:** Pay attention to which foods cause discomfort or flare-ups.

2. **Keep a Food Diary:** Tracking what you eat helps identify patterns between diet and symptoms.

3. **Eat Small Meals Frequently:** Instead of large meals that might overwhelm your digestive system, smaller meals spaced out throughout the day can be gentler.

4. **Stay Hydrated:** Diarrhea is common with Crohn's, leading to dehydration—so drinking plenty of fluids is key.

5. **Balanced Nutrition**: Ensuring you're getting enough proteins, vitamins, and minerals even on your 'safe food' list can sometimes require careful planning or supplements.

Recent Research Insights

There's some hopeful news coming from recent research on Crohn's disease! Keeping up with scientific insights really helps us feel more connected to the community striving towards better treatments.

1. **Microbiome Studies:** Researchers are diving deep into understanding our gut bacteria—the microbiome—because imbalance here is linked to Crohn's flares. Studies are suggesting that modifying gut bacteria through diet or probiotics could be beneficial.

2. **Genetic Research:** Scientists have identified over 200 genes associated with Crohn's! This isn't just fascinating—it means personalized medicine is becoming more achievable. The idea is that one day, treatments could be customized based on individual genetic makeup.

3. **Biologic Therapies:** There are new biologic drugs being developed which target specific pathways involved in inflammation more precisely than ever before, with fewer side effects compared to traditional methods.

4. **Fecal Microbiota Transplant (FMT):** Though it sounds a bit out there, FMT involves transplanting stool from a healthy donor into a Crohn's patient to reset their gut flora. It's showing promise for some patients!

5. **Stem Cell Therapy:** There are exciting advancements here too! Stem cells have the potential to repair damaged tissues and modulate immune responses more effectively. Clinical trials are ongoing but seeing positive results so far.

CHAPTER 2

Nutritional Foundations for Crohn's

Nutrients Important for Crohn's

Getting the right nutrients is essential for everyone, but it's especially crucial if you have Crohn's Disease. Your digestive system can be compromised, making it harder for your body to absorb the vitamins and minerals it needs. Proper nutrition can help manage symptoms and even reduce the frequency of flare-ups.

1. **Protein:** When battling inflammation and potential muscle loss, protein is crucial. It helps repair tissues and supports your immune system. You can find good sources in lean meats, fish, eggs, and dairy products if you can tolerate them.

2. Iron: Often people with Crohn's suffer from anemia due to bleeding or poor absorption of iron. Include iron-rich foods like lean red meat, poultry, fish, beans, lentils, and fortified cereals in your diet. Just be mindful of how well you tolerate these foods.

3. Calcium: Some medications and reduced dairy intake can affect calcium levels. Including low-fat milk, yogurt if tolerated, or alternatives like calcium-fortified plant-based milks can support bone health.

4. Vitamin D: This vitamin works hand-in-hand with calcium to maintain bone strength and reduce inflammation. Exposure to sunlight helps produce Vitamin D but also consider foods like fatty fish and fortified products.

5. Vitamin B12: Since Crohn's can affect the end of the small intestine where B12 is absorbed, it's essential to keep an eye on this vitamin. Find it in animal products or fortified cereals.

6. Folate (Vitamin B9): Necessary for red blood cell formation, folate can be found in leafy greens, legumes, and fortified grains.

NUTRIENT	ROLE	FOOD SOURCES
Protein	Tissue repair	Lean meats, fish, eggs, dairy
Iron	Prevents anemia	Red meat, poultry, fish, beans
Calcium	Bone health	Low-fat milk/yogurt, fortified plant milk
Vitamin D	Reduces inflammation	Fatty fish, fortified foods
Vitamin B12	Nerve function	Animal products, fortified cereals
Folate	Red blood cell formation	Leafy greens, legumes

Foods To Include And Avoid

Now let's discuss food choices — what should we eat more of and what might be best to leave off the plate?

Foods to Include

1. **Low-Fiber Fruits and Vegetables:** These can be easier on your system and less likely to cause irritation. Think bananas, well-cooked carrots, and peeled apples.

2. **Lean Proteins:** As we mentioned before, lean meats, fish, eggs, and tofu are good choices. They provide the necessary protein without too much fat that might aggravate symptoms.

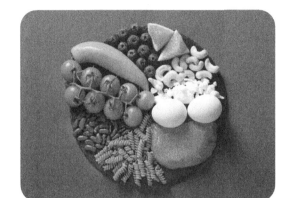

3. **Refined Grains:** While whole grains are generally healthy, their high fiber content can sometimes cause issues. Instead, opt for white bread, pasta, and rice.

4. **Lactose-Free Dairy or Alternatives:** If you find dairy hard to digest, try lactose-free options or plant-based milk like almond or rice milk.

5. **Smooth Nut Butters:** Peanut butter or almond butter can be easier to digest than whole nuts. Make sure they don't have added sugar or oils.

FOOD TYPE	WHY IT'S GOOD	EXAMPLES
Low-Fiber Fruits/Veggies	Easier on digestion	Bananas, cooked carrots, peeled apples
Lean Proteins	Provides necessary protein without high fat	Lean meats, fish, eggs, tofu
Refined Grains	Less irritating for the gut	White bread, pasta, rice
Lactose-Free Dairy/Alts	Easier digestion	Lactose-free milk/yogurt, almond milk
Smooth Nut Butters	Easier to digest than whole nuts	Peanut butter (without added sugar/oils)

Foods to Avoid

1. **High-Fiber Foods:** These can lead to more digestive discomfort or blockages. It includes raw veggies with skins, seeds, and fibrous fruits like oranges.

2. **Fatty Foods:** They may be tough on your digestive tract and can trigger symptoms. So keep fried foods and fatty cuts of meat at bay.

3. **Dairy Products:** If you're lactose intolerant or sensitive to dairy, milk and cheese can cause bloating and discomfort.

4. **Whole Nuts and Seeds:** These are hard to digest and can irritate the gut lining; instead opt for their smoother counterparts like butters.

FOOD TYPE	REASON TO AVOID	EXAMPLES
High-Fiber Foods	Can cause discomfort/blockages	Raw veggies with skins, fibrous fruits
Fatty Foods	Triggering symptoms	Fried foods, fatty cuts of meat
Dairy Products	Causes bloating if sensitive	Milk, cheese
Whole Nuts/Seeds	Hard to digest	Almonds (whole), sunflower seeds

Remember, everyone's experience with Crohn's is different. It's always a good idea to keep track of what works for you and chat with your healthcare provider about tailoring a diet that fits your needs best.

Managing Nutritional Deficiencies

Living with Crohn's means being extra mindful of potential nutritional deficiencies. The inflammation and damage caused by the disease can hinder your body's ability to absorb essential nutrients, leading to various deficiencies. Proper nutrition management is vital in keeping symptoms in check and promoting overall health.

1. **Iron:** loss from intestinal bleeding and poor absorption can lead to anemia. Incorporating iron-rich foods like lean red meats, poultry, fish, beans, lentils, and iron-fortified cereals can help.

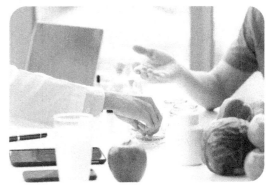

2. **Vitamin B12:** Absorption of this crucial vitamin often takes place at the end of the small intestine—an area commonly affected by Crohn's. Deficiency can lead to anemia and neurological issues. Found in animal products like meats, eggs, dairy, and fortified cereals, you might also need supplements if your levels are particularly low.

3. **Folate (Vitamin B9):** Folate is critical for cell growth and red blood cell formation. It's commonly found in leafy green vegetables, legumes, and fortified grains. If you have a deficiency, it can exacerbate anemia and other issues.

4. **Calcium:** Bone health can be an issue due to reduced dairy intake or medications like corticosteroids that impact calcium levels. Low-fat dairy products or calcium-fortified plant-based alternatives can help maintain adequate calcium levels.

5. **Magnesium:** This mineral is important in muscle function and bone health but may be deficient due to chronic diarrhea or poor absorption. Foods like nuts, seeds, whole grains, and leafy greens are good sources of magnesium.

How Do We Manage These Deficiencies?

1. **Diet Adjustments:** Incorporating foods rich in these vitamins and minerals is crucial. For instance, lean meats or spinach for iron, dairy or fortified juices for calcium, and fish or fortified cereals for vitamin D.

2. **Supplements:** Sometimes food alone can't cover the gaps. Simple supplements like a multivitamin might be necessary.

3. **Monitor Levels:** Regular blood tests help keep an eye on our nutrient levels.

4. **Work With a Dietitian:** A professional can help tailor your diet specifically to your needs.

Hydration and Digestive Health

When it comes to managing Crohn's Disease effectively, hydration plays an unsung hero role that cannot be overstated. Proper hydration aids digestion and nutrient absorption and helps maintain overall well-being. You might not think about water when planning your diet for Crohn's Disease but staying hydrated is crucial:

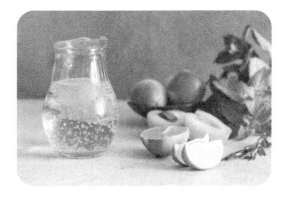

1. **Digestive Function:** Water aids in breaking down

food so that your body can absorb the nutrients.

2. **Flushing Out Toxins:** Staying hydrated helps flush out waste products through urine.

3. **Medication Efficacy:** Many medications for Crohn's Disease need adequate fluid intake to work effectively.

4. **Preventing Dehydration:** Symptoms like diarrhea can cause rapid fluid loss leading to dehydration.

Tips for Staying Hydrated

1. Aim for at least 8-10 glasses of water a day but adjust based on your individual needs.

2. Keep an eye on urine color; pale yellow is generally an indication of good hydration.

3. Include water-rich foods like cucumbers, watermelon, oranges, grapefruit, strawberries, lettuce, zucchini.

Beyond plain water though:

1. **Broths/soups:** Great dual benefit — hydrating while also being gentle on the stomach.

2. **Herbal teas:** Add variety but avoid caffeinated options since caffeine can worsen dehydration.

3. **Electrolyte drinks:** Especially after bouts of diarrhea; these helps replenish lost minerals like sodium/potassium quickly.

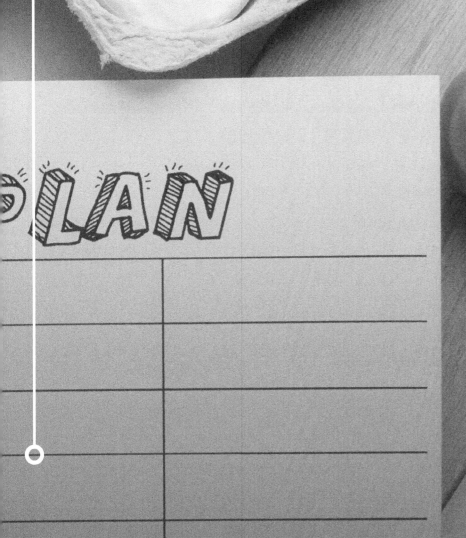

CHAPTER 3

THE 28-DAY MEAL PLAN

Daily Meal Breakdowns
— — — · · ·

DAY	BREAKFAST	LUNCH	DINNER	DESSERTS
			WEEK 1	
1	Mango Chia Seed Pudding	Spinach and Potato Frittata	Lentil and Kale Stew	Pumpkin Rice Pudding
2	Avocado and Egg White Omelette	Turkey Meatball Zoodles	Baked Zucchini Boats	Lemon Vanilla Rice Balls
3	Cottage Cheese with Melon Slices	Shrimp & Avocado Rice Bowl	Lemon Herb Chicken Breast	Fig and Date Energy Balls
4	Greek Yogurt with Honey and Blueberries	Roasted Beet Salad	Greek Yogurt Chicken Salad	Soft Pumpkin Bars
5	Soft-Boiled Eggs with Toast	Cauliflower Rice with Turmeric	Baked Tilapia with Asparagus	Tapioca Pudding
6	Banana Oatmeal Smoothie	Steamed Cod with Ginger	Lentil and Vegetable Patties	Sautéed Cinnamon Apples
7	Scrambled Eggs with Spinach	Chicken and Brown Rice Soup	Gentle Sauteed Spinach and Turkey	Soft Peanut Butter Cookies
WEEK 2				
8	Carrot and Ginger Juice Smoothie	Carrot and Hummus Wrap	Grilled Turkey Tenderloins with Herbs	Peach Yogurt Popsicles
9	Fluffy Coconut Flour Pancakes	Brown Rice and Broccoli Bowl	Oven-Baked Herb-Crusted Tilapia	Silken Tofu Chocolate Mousse

DAY	BREAKFAST	LUNCH	DINNER	DESSERTS
10	Pumpkin Spice Oatmeal	Rice Paper Veggie Rolls with Peanut Sauce	Tender Baked Tofu Stir-Fry	Rice Flour Crepes with Berry Compote
11	Soft Boiled Eggs on Asparagus Tips	Soft Tofu Veggie Stir-Fry	Lemon Dill Poached Chicken	Strawberry Banana Sorbet
12	Chicken and Rice Porridge	Coconut Rice with Steamed Vegetables	Nourishing Chicken Broth with Noodles	Gingerbread Loaf
13	Buckwheat Pancakes with Maple Syrup	Grilled Salmon with Asparagus	Delicate Sweet Potato Rice Bowl	Applesauce Cupcakes
14	Low-Fat Ricotta on Whole Grain Bread	Pineapple Chicken Skewers	Spinach and Ricotta Stuffed Mushrooms	Sweet Potato Pudding
WEEK 3				
15	Quinoa Breakfast Bowls with Berries	Roasted Butternut Squash Soup	Savory Turkey Burgers	Almond Milk Ice Cream
16	Soft Polenta with Steamed Vegetables	Tomato Basil Soup with Grilled Zucchini	Carrot and Ginger Salmon Patties	Raspberry Oat Bars
17	Berry Smoothie Bowl	Turkey and Spinach Lettuce Wraps	Gentle Chicken Stew	Coconut Macaroons
18	Sweet Potato Hash Browns	Zucchini Noodles with Marinara Sauce	Soft-Baked Tilapia Fillets	Creamy Avocado Pudding
19	Vegetable and Quinoa Frittata	Turkey and Quinoa Vegetable Stir-Fry	Broiled Lemon Herb Shrimp	Coconut Water Jello Cubes

DAY	BREAKFAST	LUNCH	DINNER	DESSERTS
20	Almond Butter Banana Toast	Ginger Carrot Soup	Black Bean Quinoa-Stuffed Bell Peppers	Lemon Gelatin Dessert
21	Millet Porridge with Cinnamon	Grilled Chicken and Avocado Salad	Mild Beef Stew	Pumpkin Rice Pudding
WEEK 4				
22	Poached Salmon on Toast	Steamed Tilapia with Lemon and Dill	Grilled Mahi-Mahi with Mango Salsa	Lemon Vanilla Rice Balls
23	Soft Tofu Scramble with Herbs	Lentil and Quinoa Stuffed Peppers	Gentle Fish Tacos	Fig and Date Energy Balls
24	Applesauce Muffins	Poached Chicken Slaw	Baked Cod with Vegetables	Soft Pumpkin Bars
25	Gluten-Free Waffles with Bananas	Brown Rice Avocado Sushi Rolls	Steamed Veggie Medley	Tapioca Pudding
26	Mango Chia Seed Pudding	Spinach and Potato Frittata	Lentil and Kale Stew	Sautéed Cinnamon Apples
27	Avocado and Egg White Omelette	Turkey Meatball Zoodles	Baked Zucchini Boats	Soft Peanut Butter Cookies
28	Cottage Cheese with Melon Slices	Shrimp & Avocado Rice Bowl	Lemon Herb Chicken Breast	Peach Yogurt Popsicles

Nutritional Goals for Each Week

When it comes to managing Crohn's Disease through diet, consistency is key. What we eat has a profound impact on our gut health, energy levels, and overall well-being. The journey might seem overwhelming at first, but by approaching it week-by-week, nutritional goals can become more manageable. Here's a simple guide to help you navigate your meals and make choices that nurture your body.

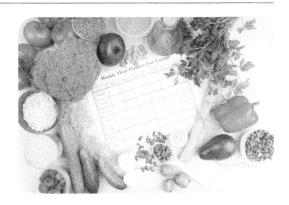

Week 1: Hydration and Soft Foods

The first week is all about easing into changes. Let's start with hydration because it's critical for digestion and healing.

Hydration Targets:

- ✔ Aim for at least 8 cups of fluids daily. This can include water, herbal teas, and clear broths.
- ✔ Avoid caffeinated drinks which can irritate the digestive system.

Soft Food Choices:

- ✔ Focus on gentle foods like bananas, applesauce, and well-cooked vegetables.
- ✔ Include plain rice, oatmeal, and tender proteins such as poached chicken or fish.

Week 2: Introducing Probiotics

In the second week, we're introducing foods that are good for gut health. Probiotics are beneficial bacteria that can improve digestion and reduce inflammation.

Probiotic Foods:

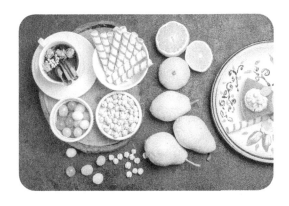

- ✔ Try yogurt with live cultures (if you tolerate dairy).
- ✔ Kefir is another excellent option—it's a fermented drink full of probiotics.
- ✔ Miso soup made with low-sodium broth can also be included.

Still Keep It Gentle:

- ✔ Continue with the soft foods from week one.

- ✔ Make sure to listen to your body—if something feels off, adjust accordingly.

Week 3: Fiber in Moderation

Fiber is essential for digestive health but too much can be problematic. This week is about finding a balance.

Soluble Fiber Sources:

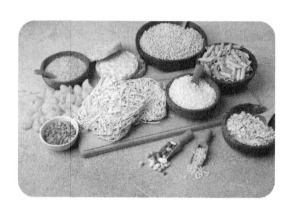

- ✔ Oats, peeled apples (cooked), carrots, and squash are great options.

- ✔ Consider incorporating chia seeds into smoothies or yogurt for added soluble fiber.

Avoid Insoluble Fibers:

- ✔ Steer clear of raw vegetables, nuts, seeds (except chia), and whole grains which might be too harsh on the gut.

Week 4: Healthy Fats

Fat is necessary for energy and nutrient absorption. Choosing the right kind will benefit your gut.

Healthy Fat Sources:

- ✔ Avocados are packed with healthy fats and gentle on the digestive system.
- ✔ Olive oil is great for cooking or drizzling over steamed vegetables.
- ✔ Fatty fish like salmon provide omega-3 fatty acids which reduce inflammation.

Tips for Meal Prep

With a bit of planning, meal prep can make a world of difference. Prepping meals in advance ensures you always have something safe and nutritious on hand, reduces the stress of last-minute cooking, and helps avoid those quick, unhealthy options that might trigger a flare-up.

One of the first steps is to create a clean and organized kitchen. Make sure to stock up on your safe and favorite ingredients—those that you know don't trigger symptoms. Having a well-organized pantry and refrigerator makes it easier to find everything you need when it's time to cook.

Think about investing in some good quality storage containers. Glass containers with airtight lids are great because they keep your food fresh and are microwave-safe—perfect for reheating. Label each container with the date and contents so you always know what's inside and when it was made.

Try to choose recipes that can be made in bulk and frozen for later use. Soups, stews, and casseroles are all excellent choices because they reheat well and often taste even better after the flavors have had time to meld together. On weekends or days when you feel better, cook larger batches of these meals, portion them out, and freeze them.

When you're making meals ahead of time, balance is key. Your body needs a variety of nutrients to stay healthy, especially when managing a chronic condition like Crohn's Disease. Focus on incorporating lean proteins, easily digestible carbohydrates like white rice or potatoes, healthy fats like olive oil or avocado, and cooked fruits and vegetables.

Always listen to your body. What works for one person with Crohn's may not work for another. Keep track of what you eat in a food diary—noting not just what you ate but how you felt afterward. Over time, you'll identify patterns that will help you make smarter choices about meal prep.

Lastly, let's not forget hydration. Always have a bottle of water handy to keep yourself hydrated throughout the day. Herbal teas can also be a soothing option—just steer clear of any that might irritate your system.

Adjusting the Plan for Flare-Ups

Even with careful planning and the best preventive measures, flare-ups can still happen. It's essential to have a flexible approach when they do.

During a flare-up, your body might be more sensitive than usual, necessitating gentle adjustments in what you eat. The goal is to minimize irritation while ensuring nutritional needs are met.

Opt for bland foods that are easy on the stomach. These might include things like plain toast (white bread), plain pasta or noodles (again without whole grains), boiled potatoes without skin, scrambled eggs, or smooth peanut butter (if tolerated). Remember the BRAT diet—Bananas, Rice, Applesauce, Toast—which is often effective during gastrointestinal distress.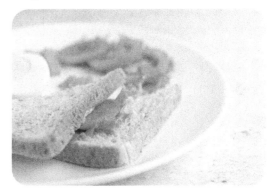

Stick with soft, cooked vegetables as opposed to raw ones since they're easier to digest. Pureeing soups or stews can make them easier on your digestive system while still providing good nutrition.

Keep an easy-to-digest protein source handy like poached chicken or mild fish such as cod or sole—these are less likely to upset your stomach compared to stronger flavored.

Also, it's okay to cut back on fiber temporarily. Fiber can be harsh during flare-ups, so opt for white bread instead of whole grain bread and well-cooked vegetables rather than salads.

Hydration becomes even more crucial during a flare-up. Dehydration can make symptoms worse, so sip on fluids throughout the day. Oral rehydration solutions can help maintain electrolyte balance. Gentle options like broth or diluted juices can also be soothing. It's beneficial to prepare some *"flare-up friendly"* meals ahead of time and keep them in the freezer. This way, if you don't feel up to cooking, you still have easy access to safe meals.

SAFE DURING FLARE-UPS	FOODS TO AVOID DURING FLARE-UPS
Plain toast (white bread)	Whole grain bread
Plain pasta	Spicy foods
Boiled potatoes	Raw vegetables
Scrambled eggs	High-fiber fruits like berries or apples
Smooth peanut butter	Seeds and nuts
Poached chicken	Fatty cuts of meat

Remember, it's essential to communicate with your healthcare provider about any diet changes, especially during flare-ups. They'll be able to provide tailored advice based on your specific needs.

CHAPTER 4

RECIPE SECTION

Breakfasts

1. Mango Chia Seed Pudding

Prep time:
15 mins

Cooking time:
N/A

Servings:
4

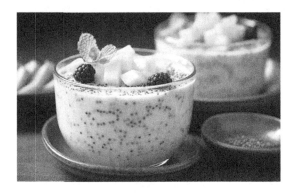

Ingredients:

- One cup mango puree
- Two tbsp chia seeds
- One cup almond milk
- Two tbsp unsweetened coconut flakes

Tips: For extra texture, mix in some pieces of fresh mango before serving.

Serving size: 1 cup

Nutritional values (per serving): Calories: 120; Fat: 4g; Carbs: 18g; Protein: 2g; Sodium: 40mg; Sugar: 12g; Cholesterol: 0mg; Fiber: 3g

Directions:

1. In your container, mix mango puree, and milk. Mix in chia seeds. Pour it into serving cups or bowls.
2. Let it sit in your refrigerator for at least four hours. Before serving, top with coconut flakes.

2. Quinoa Breakfast Bowls with Berries

Prep time:
10 mins

Cooking time:
15

Servings:
4

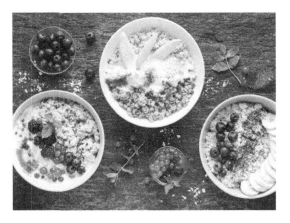

Ingredients:

- One cup quinoa, washed
- Two cups water
- One cup mixed berries
- Two tbsp honey
- One tsp vanilla extract

Tips: Feel free to swap out mixed berries for any single type of berry or other soft fruit.

Serving size: 1 bowl

Nutritional values (per serving): Calories: 225; Fat: 5g; Carbs: 40g; Protein: 7g; Sodium: 25mg; Sugar: 14g; Cholesterol: 0mg; Fiber: 5g

Directions:

1. In your medium pot, let water boil, then add the quinoa. Adjust to low temp, cover, then simmer for fifteen mins till quinoa is fluffy.
2. In your container, mix cooked quinoa with honey and vanilla. Divide it into four bowls. Top each with mixed berries.

3. Applesauce Muffins

Prep time: 10 mins

Cooking time: 20 mins

Servings: 12

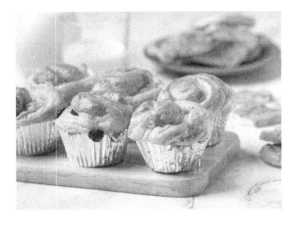

Ingredients:

- Two cups whole wheat flour
- One tsp baking soda
- Half tsp cinnamon
- One cup unsweetened apple-sauce
- Half cup maple syrup
- Quarter cup vegetable oil

Tips: Ensure the muffins are completely cooled before consuming to avoid any potential gastrointestinal irritation.

Serving size: One muffin

Nutritional values (per serving): Calories: 150; Fat: 6g; Carbs: 24g; Protein: 2g; Sodium: 180mg; Sugar: 12g; Cholesterol: 0mg; Fiber: 3g

Directions:

1. Warm up your oven to 350°F (177°C).
2. In your big container, whisk flour, baking soda and cinnamon.
3. In another container, mix applesauce, syrup, and oil. Slowly add the wet mixture in it while mixing.
4. Pour it into your lined muffin tin, then bake for twenty mins till golden brown.

4. Gluten-Free Waffles With Bananas

Prep time: 10 mins

Cooking time: 15 mins

Servings: 4

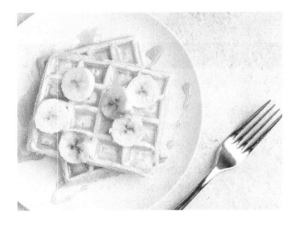

Ingredients:

- One & half cups gluten-free flour mix
- One tbsp baking powder
- One tbsp sugar
- One cup almond milk
- Two big eggs
- Two ripe bananas, mashed
- One tbsp olive oil

Tips: Make sure to mash bananas well to integrate smoothly into the batter.

Serving size: One waffle

Nutritional values (per serving): Calories: 255; Fat: 8g; Carbs: 41g; Protein: 6g; Sodium: 300mg; Sugar: 12g; Cholesterol: 55mg; Fiber: 3g

Directions:

1. In your big container, mix flour, baking powder, and sugar.
2. In another container, whisk milk, eggs, bananas, and olive oil. Combine it with flour mixture till blended.
3. Warm up your waffle iron, then lightly grease it with oil. Pour the batter into your waffle iron and cook for three mins till golden brown.

5. Soft Tofu Scramble with Herbs

Prep time: 5 mins   **Cooking time:** 10 mins   **Servings:** 2

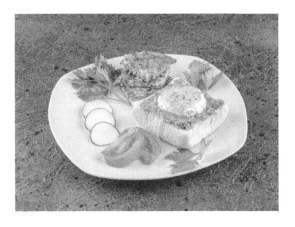

Ingredients:

- One lb. soft tofu, strained & crumbled
- Two tbsp nutritional yeast
- One tbsp olive oil
- One tsp turmeric powder
- Salt, as required
- Two tbsp parsley or basil, chopped
- One tsp powdered garlic

Tips: Serve with gluten-free toast or a side salad for a more complete meal.

Serving size: Half lb. tofu scramble

Nutritional values (per serving): Calories: 185; Fat: 10g; Carbs: 9g; Protein: 16g; Sodium: 320mg; Sugar: 2g; Cholesterol: 0mg; Fiber: 3g

Directions:

1. Warm up oil in your non-stick skillet on moderate temp. Add crumbled tofu, then mix for two mins.
2. Sprinkle in nutritional yeast, turmeric, powdered garlic, and salt, then mix well. Continue cooking for five more mins till the tofu is slightly golden.
3. Remove, then mix in fresh herbs before serving.

6. Poached Salmon on Toast

Prep time: 15 mins   **Cooking time:** 10 mins   **Servings:** 2

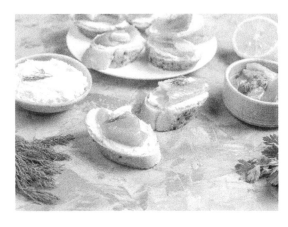

Ingredients:

- Two salmon fillets (about one lb. total)
- Two cups of water
- One tbsp lemon juice
- One tsp dried dill
- Salt, as required
- Four slices of whole-grain bread, toasted

Tips: Use fresh dill if available for added flavor.

Serving size: 1 slice with salmon

Nutritional values (per serving): Calories: 280; Fat: 12g; Carbs: 18g; Protein: 24g; Sodium: 400mg; Sugar: 2g; Cholesterol: 60mg; Fiber: 3g

Directions:

1. In your big skillet, let water, lemon juice, dill, and salt simmer. Add salmon fillets and poach for ten mins till fish flakes easily.
2. Put salmon onto your toasted bread slices. Serve.

7. Millet Porridge with Cinnamon

Prep time:	Cooking time:	Servings:
5 mins	15 mins	4

Ingredients:

- One cup millet, washed
- Three cups of water
- One tsp cinnamon powder
- A pinch of salt

Tips: Garnish with fresh berries or a sprinkle of nuts for added nutrition.

Serving size: 1 cup

Nutritional values (per serving): Calories: 145; Fat: 2g; Carbs: 28g; Protein: 4g; Sodium: 30mg; Sugar: 6g; Cholesterol: 0mg; Fiber: 3g

Directions:

1. In your medium saucepan, mix millet, water, cinnamon, and salt.
2. Let it boil, then simmer for fifteen mins till millet is tender. Serve warm.

8. Almond Butter Banana Toast

Prep time:	Cooking time:	Servings:
5 mins	N/A	1

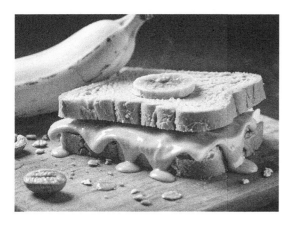

Ingredients:

- One slice whole grain bread, toasted
- One tbsp almond butter
- Half a banana, thinly sliced

Tips: Use gluten-free bread if you are sensitive to gluten.

Serving size: 1 piece of toast

Nutritional values (per serving): Calories: 220; Fat: 10g; Carbs: 28g; Protein: 6g; Sodium: 110mg; Sugar: 13g; Cholesterol: 0mg; Fiber: 4g

Directions:

1. Spread the almond butter evenly over your toast.
2. Arrange the banana slices on top of the almond butter. Serve.

9. Vegetable and Quinoa Frittata

Prep time: 10 mins **Cooking time:** 15 mins **Servings:** 4

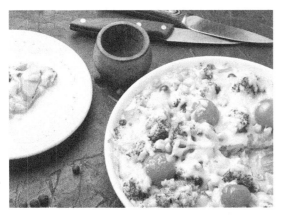

Ingredients:

- Six big eggs
- Half cup cooked quinoa
- Half cup spinach, chopped
- One tomato, diced
- One small zucchini, diced
- One tbsp olive oil
- Salt, as required

Tips: Can be enjoyed warm or cold.

Serving size: 1 slice (one-fourth of frittata)

Nutritional values (per serving): Calories: 290; Fat: 19g; Carbs: 10g; Protein: 16g; Sodium: 260mg; Sugar: 2g; Cholesterol: 310mg; Fiber: 2g

Directions:

1. Warm up your oven to 350°F (177°C).
2. In your medium container, beat eggs, then flavor it with salt. Mix in cooked quinoa, spinach, tomato, and zucchini.
3. Warm up oil in your non-stick skillet on moderate temp. Pour egg mixture into your skillet, then cook for three mins, till edges start to set.
4. Transfer skillet to your oven, then bake for twelve mins till fully set.

10. Sweet Potato Hash Browns

Prep time: 15 mins **Cooking time:** 15 mins **Servings:** 4

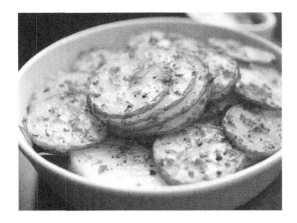

Ingredients:

- Two medium sweet potatoes, peeled & grated
- One tbsp olive oil
- One tsp salt
- One tsp black pepper
- One tsp smoked paprika

Tips: Serve with a side of avocado or a dollop of Greek yogurt for added flavor.

Serving size: 1 hash brown patty

Nutritional values (per serving): Calories: 80; Fat: 3g; Carbs: 12g; Protein: 1g; Sodium: 200mg; Sugar: 2g; Cholesterol: 0mg; Fiber: 2g

Directions:

1. Warm up oil in your big non-stick skillet on moderate temp.
2. In your container, mix sweet potatoes, salt, pepper, and paprika. Form it into small patties.
3. Cook patties in your skillet for four to five mins per side till golden. Serve.

Lunches

11. Spinach And Potato Frittata

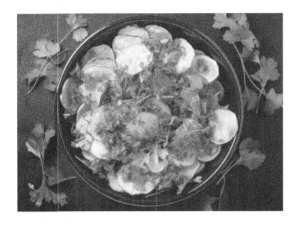

Prep time: 10 mins

Cooking time: 20 mins

Servings: 4

Ingredients:

- One tbsp olive oil
- One cup baby spinach
- Two medium potatoes, thinly sliced
- Six big eggs
- One fourth cup milk
- One tsp salt
- Half tsp black pepper

Tips: Ensure potatoes are thinly sliced for quicker cooking.

Serving size: 1 slice (one fourth of frittata)

Nutritional values (per serving): Calories: 150; Fat: 8g; Carbs: 12g; Protein: 8g; Sodium: 300mg; Sugar: 2g; Cholesterol: 170mg; Fiber: 2g

Directions:

1. Warm up your oven to 350°F (177° C). Warm up oil in your oven-safe skillet on moderate temp.
2. Add potatoes, then cook for five to seven mins till tender. Add spinach, then cook for two mins till wilted.
3. Whisk eggs, milk, salt, and pepper in your container. Pour it over your potatoes and spinach. Cook for three to four mins till edges are set.
4. Transfer skillet to your oven, then bake for ten mins till the center is set.

12. Brown Rice Avocado Sushi Rolls

Prep time: 20 mins

Cooking time: 40 mins

Servings: 4

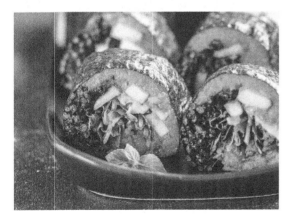

Ingredients:

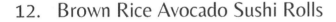

- Two cups cooked brown rice
- Two tbsp rice vinegar
- One tbsp sugar
- One tsp salt
- Two avocados, sliced
- Four sheets nori (seaweed)
- One cucumber, juliennedd

Tips: Use a wet knife to cut the rolls cleanly.

Serving size: Two rolls

Nutritional values (per serving): Calories: 220; Fat: 10g; Carbs: 32g; Protein: 4g; Sodium: 225mg; Sugar: 2g; Cholesterol: 0mg; Fiber: 7g

Directions:

5. Mix zzzzrice vinegar, sugar, and salt into the cooked brown rice. Place a nori sheet on your bamboo sushi mat.
6. Spread some seasoned brown rice over your nori. Arrange avocado and cucumber slices horizontally across the middle of your rice.
7. Roll the bamboo mat away from you pressing gently to form a tight roll. Cut into bite-sized pieces.

13. Tomato Basil Soup With Grilled Zucchini

Prep time: 15 mins

Cooking time: 30 mins

Servings: 4

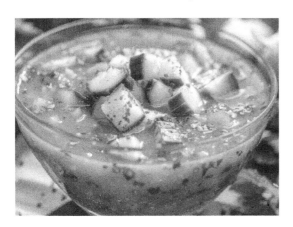

Ingredients:

- Six cups diced tomatoes (canned or fresh)
- Two cups vegetable broth (low-sodium)
- One tbsp olive oil
- One cup basil leaves, chopped
- One cup diced zucchini
- One tsp dried oregano
- Salt & pepper, as required

Tips: Pair with gluten-free bread for a complete meal.

Serving size: 1 & 1/2 cups of soup + 1/4 cup of grilled zucchini

Nutritional values (per serving): Calories: 110; Fat: 5g; Carbs: 16g; Protein: 2g; Sodium: 320mg; Sugar: 8g; Cholesterol: 0mg; Fiber: 3g

Directions:

1. In your big pot, warm up oil on moderate temp. Add tomatoes and broth, then let it simmer. Add basil leaves and oregano, continue to simmer for twenty mins.
2. Grill zucchini on a grill pan till tender and slightly charred. Blend soup till smooth, then flavor it with salt and pepper. Serve hot with grilled zucchini slices on top.

14. Poached Chicken Slaw

Prep time: 15 mins

Cooking time: 20 mins

Servings: 4

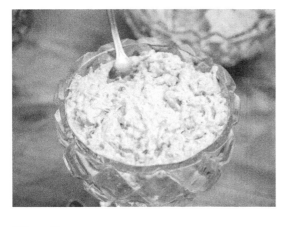

Ingredients:

- Two chicken breasts (about one lb.)
- Two cups shredded cabbage
- One cup grated carrots
- One apple, thinly sliced
- Two tbsp olive oil
- One tbsp apple cider vinegar
- One tsp honey
- Salt & pepper, as required

Tips: Serve with a side of fresh fruit for added nutrients.

Serving size: 1 cup

Nutritional values (per serving): Calories: 250; Fat: 7g; Carbs: 22g; Protein: 24g; Sodium: 300mg; Sugar: 12g; Cholesterol: 50mg; Fiber: 3g

Directions:

1. Poach the chicken breasts in boiling water for ten to fifteen mins, till fully cooked. Let the chicken cool, then shred it with a fork.
2. In your big container, mix cabbage, carrots, and apple. In your small container, whisk oil, apple cider, honey, salt, and pepper.
3. Toss the chicken and dressing with the slaw mixture. Chill in the refrigerator before serving.

15. Lentil And Quinoa Stuffed Peppers

Prep time: 15 mins   **Cooking time:** 35 mins   **Servings:** 4

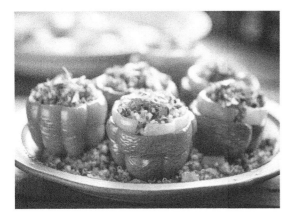

Ingredients:

- Four bell peppers, top cut off and seeds removed
- One cup cooked quinoa
- One cup cooked lentils
- Half lb. ground turkey breast (optional)
- One cup diced tomatoes
- One tsp cumin
- Two tbsp olive oil
- Salt & pepper, as required

Tips: Use different colored bell peppers for variety in presentation.

Serving size: 1 stuffed pepper

Nutritional values (per serving): Calories: 300; Fat: 8g; Carbs: 35g; Protein: 21g; Sodium: 400mg; Sugar: 7g; Cholesterol: 50mg; Fiber: 8g

Directions:

1. Warm up your oven to 375°F (190°C). If using turkey, cook it in a pan on moderate temp till browned.
2. In your container, mix quinoa, lentils, tomatoes, cumin, olive oil, salt, and pepper. Add cooked turkey if desired. Stuff each bell pepper with it.
3. Put stuffed peppers in your baking dish, then cover using aluminum foil. Bake for thirty to thirty-five mins or till peppers are tender.

16. Steamed Tilapia with Lemon and Dill

Prep time: 10 mins   **Cooking time:** 15 mins   **Servings:** 4

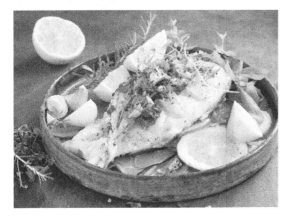

Ingredients:

- Four tilapia fillets
- One lemon, sliced
- One tsp dried dill
- One tbsp olive oil
- Salt & pepper, as required

Tips: Serve with a side of steamed vegetables or a light salad for a balanced meal.

Serving size: 1 fillet

Nutritional values (per serving): Calories: 150; Fat: 5g; Carbs: 2g; Protein: 25g; Sodium: 50mg; Sugar: 0g; Cholesterol: 55mg; Fiber: 0g

Directions:

1. Flavor tilapia fillets with salt, pepper, and dried dill. Place lemon slices evenly on each fillet.
2. Drizzle olive oil over the fillets. Steam for fifteen mins till fish flakes easily.

17. Grilled Chicken And Avocado Salad

 Prep time: 15 mins

 Cooking time: 10 mins

 Servings: 4

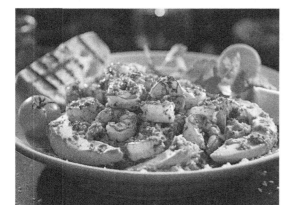

Ingredients:

- Two grilled chicken breasts, sliced
- Two avocados, diced
- Four cups mixed salad greens
- One cup cherry tomatoes, halved
- One cucumber, sliced
- Two tbsp olive oil
- One tbsp lemon juice
- Salt & pepper, as required

Tips: Add a sprinkle of sunflower seeds for extra crunch.

Serving size: 1/4 of salad

Nutritional values (per serving): Calories: 290; Fat: 21g; Carbs: 11g; Protein: 24g; Sodium: 60mg; Sugar: 3g; Cholesterol: 65mg; Fiber: 7g

Directions:

1. In your big container, mix salad greens, tomatoes, cucumber, and avocado. Top it with chicken slices.
2. Drizzle with olive oil and lemon juice. Flavor it with salt and pepper.

18. Ginger Carrot Soup

 Prep time: 10 mins

 Cooking time: 20 mins

 Servings: 4

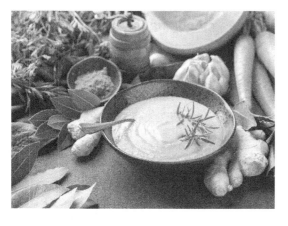

Ingredients:

- One lb. carrots, peeled and chopped
- Three cups low-sodium vegetable broth
- One tbsp ginger, grated
- One cup coconut milk
- One tbsp olive oil
- Salt & pepper, as required

Tips: For extra flavor, garnish with fresh parsley or cilantro.

Serving size: 1 cup

Nutritional values (per serving): Calories: 120; Fat: 7g; Carbs: 12g; Protein: 2g; Sodium: 180mg; Sugar: 6g; Cholesterol: 0mg; Fiber: 3g

Directions:

1. Warm up oil in your big pot on moderate temp. Add carrots and ginger, then sauté for five mins.
2. Pour in broth, then let it boil. Simmer for ten to fifteen mins till carrots are tender. Mix in coconut milk, then flavor it with salt and pepper.
3. Puree the soup using your immersion blender to till smooth.

19. Turkey And Quinoa Vegetable Stir-Fry

Prep time: 15 mins

Cooking time: 15 mins

Servings: 4

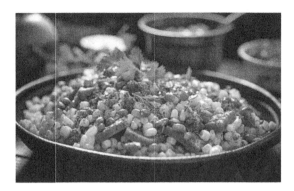

Ingredients:

- One lb. ground turkey
- One cup quinoa, cooked
- Two cups mixed vegetables (carrots, bell peppers, zucchini)
- Two tbsp soy sauce, low-sodium
- One tbsp olive oil
- Two cloves garlic, minced
- One tsp ginger, grated

Tips: Use fresh or frozen vegetables based on preference.

Serving size: 1 cup

Nutritional values (per serving): Calories: 290; Fat: 13g; Carbs: 19g; Protein: 21g; Sodium: 250mg; Sugar: 4g; Cholesterol: 70mg; Fiber: 5g

Directions:

1. Warm up oil in your big skillet on moderate-high temp. Put ground turkey, then cook till browned. Mix in garlic and ginger, then sauté for one to two mins.
2. Add mixed vegetables, then cook for four to five mins till tender. Mix in cooked quinoa and soy sauce, then cook for an additional three to four mins.

20. Zucchini Noodles With Marinara Sauce

Prep time: 15 mins

Cooking time: 10 mins

Servings: 4

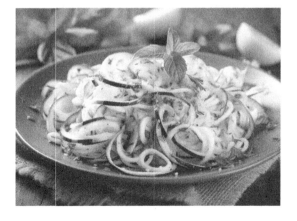

Ingredients:

- Four medium zucchini, spiralized
- One cup marinara sauce, low-sodium
- One tbsp olive oil
- Two cloves garlic, minced
- One tsp dried basil
- One tsp dried oregano
- Salt & pepper, as required

Tips: To avoid watery noodles, don't overcook the zucchini.

Serving size: 1 cup

Nutritional values (per serving): Calories: 65; Fat: 3g; Carbs: 8g; Protein: 2g; Sodium: 200mg; Sugar: 5g; Cholesterol: 0mg; Fiber: 2g

Directions:

1. Warm up oil in your big skillet on moderate temp. Add garlic and sauté for one to two mins till fragrant.
2. Add zucchini noodles, then cook for two to three mins till slightly tender.
3. Pour in the marinara sauce, dried basil, and dried oregano. Stir to mix and cook for another five mins till heated through. Flavor it with salt and pepper.

Dinners

· · ·

21. Lentil And Kale Stew

Prep time: 10 mins   **Cooking time:** 30 mins   **Servings:** 4

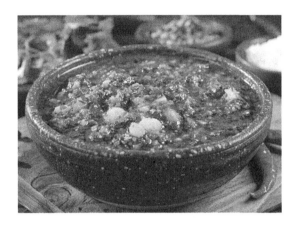

Ingredients:

- One cup dried lentils, rinsed
- Four cups low-sodium vegetable broth
- Two cups chopped kale
- One cup diced carrots
- Two tbsp olive oil
- One tsp ground turmeric
- One tsp ground cumin

Tips: Add a splash of lemon juice before serving to enhance flavor.

Serving size: 1 cup

Nutritional values (per serving): Calories: 220; Fat: 6g; Carbs: 32g; Protein: 12g; Sodium: 150mg; Sugar: 4g; Cholesterol: 0mg; Fiber: 8g

Directions:

1. In a pot, warm up oil on moderate temp. Add carrots, then cook for five mins till tender. Add lentils, broth, turmeric, and cumin. Let it boil.
2. Simmer for twenty-five mins till lentils are tender. Mix in kale, then cook for additional five mins.

22. Steamed Veggie Medley

Prep time: 10 mins   **Cooking time:** 15 mins   **Servings:** 4

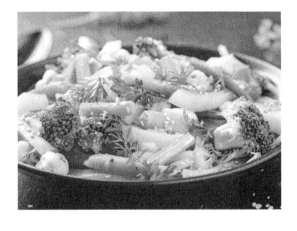

Ingredients:

- Two cups broccoli florets
- One cup baby carrots, halved
- One cup snap peas
- One tbsp olive oil
- One tsp minced garlic
- Salt, as required

Tips: You can substitute or add other vegetables like zucchini or bell peppers.

Serving size: 1 cup

Nutritional values (per serving): Calories: 45; Fat: 3g; Carbs: 8g; Protein: 2g; Sodium: 30mg; Sugar: 3g; Cholesterol: 0mg; Fiber: 3g

Directions:

1. In your big pot, add one inch of water, then let it boil. Put broccoli, carrots, and snap peas in your steamer basket on boiling water.
2. Cover, then steam for ten mins till vegetables are tender. In your pan, warm up oil on moderate temp, add garlic, then sauté for one minute.
3. Add steamed vegetables, then toss to coat in garlic and oil. Flavor it with salt, then serve.

23. Baked Cod with Vegetables

 Prep time: 10 mins

 **Cooking time:** 20 mins

 Servings: 4

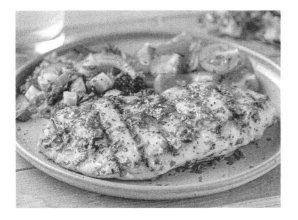

Ingredients:

- Four cod fillets (about one lb. total)
- One cup cherry tomatoes, halved
- One cup zucchini, sliced thinly
- Two tbsp olive oil
- One tsp dried oregano
- Salt & pepper, as required

Tips: For added flavor, you can drizzle lemon juice over the baked fish before serving.

Serving size: 1 fillet with vegetables

Nutritional values (per serving): Calories: 200; Fat: 8g; Carbs: 5g; Protein: 25g; Sodium: 200mg; Sugar: 3g; Cholesterol: 60mg; Fiber: 1g

Directions:

1. Warm up your oven to 400°F (204°C). Put cod fillets on your lined baking sheet. Arrange cherry tomatoes and zucchini slices around the fillets.
2. Drizzle oil over fish and vegetables, then sprinkle oregano, salt, and pepper evenly. Bake for twenty mins or till fish flakes easily.

24. Gentle Fish Tacos

 Prep time: 10 mins

 Cooking time: 15 mins

 Servings: 4

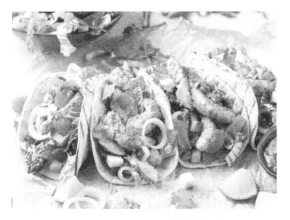

Ingredients:

- One lb. white fish (like cod or tilapia)
- One tbsp olive oil
- One tsp ground cumin
- One tsp paprika
- One tsp powdered garlic
- Eight small corn tortillas
- Half cup chopped fresh cilantro
- Juice of one lime

Tips: Serve with a side of avocado for added creaminess.

Serving size: 2 tacos

Nutritional values (per serving): Calories: 250; Fat: 7g; Carbs: 27g; Protein: 24g; Sodium: 300mg; Sugar: 2g; Cholesterol: 50mg; Fiber: 4g

1. Warm up your oven to 400°F (204°C).
2. Brush the fish with oil, then flavor it with cumin, paprika, and powdered garlic. Bake the fish for fifteen mins, till it flakes easily.
3. Warm the tortillas in a skillet on moderate temp. Flake the baked fish and distribute among the tortillas. Sprinkle cilantro on top and drizzle with lime juice.

25. Savory Turkey Burgers

Prep time: 10 mins

Cooking time: 15 mins

Servings: 4

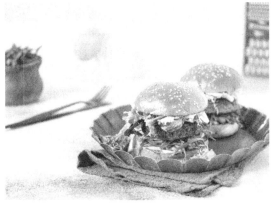

Ingredients:

- One lb. ground turkey
- One tsp powdered garlic
- One tsp dried thyme
- Half tsp sea salt
- Half cup finely chopped spinach
- One tbsp olive oil
- Whole grain burger buns (optional)

Tips: Pair with steamed vegetables or sweet potato wedges for a balanced meal.

Serving size: 1 burger

Nutritional values (per serving): Calories: 270; Fat: 12g; Carbs: 14g; Protein: 25g; Sodium: 350mg; Sugar: 2g; Cholesterol: 70mg; Fiber: 3g

Directions:

1. Warm up your grill or skillet to moderate-high temp.
2. In your container, mix ground turkey, powdered garlic, thyme, sea salt, and spinach. Form mixture into four equal patties.
3. Brush skillet or grill with olive oil and cook burgers for seven mins per side, till thoroughly cooked. Serve on whole grain buns if desired.

26. Grilled Mahi-Mahi With Mango Salsa

Prep time: 15 mins

Cooking time: 10 mins

Servings: 4

Ingredients:

- Four mahi-mahi fillets (about one lb.)
- One cup diced mango
- One-half cup diced red bell pepper
- One-fourth cup chopped red onion
- Two tbsp fresh lime juice
- Two tbsp chopped fresh cilantro
- Salt & pepper, as required

Tips: For added flavor, marinate the fillets in a simple marinade of olive oil, lime juice, and garlic before grilling.

Serving size: 1 fillet with 1/4 cup salsa

Nutritional values (per serving): Calories: 210; Fat: 3g; Carbs: 12g; Protein: 27g; Sodium: 130mg; Sugar: 9g; Cholesterol: 80mg; Fiber: 2g

Directions:

1. Warm up your grill to moderate-high temp. Flavor mahi-mahi fillets with salt and pepper. Grill the fillets for four to five mins on each side till cooked through.
2. In your container, mix mango, bell pepper, onion, lime juice, cilantro, and salt. Serve the grilled mahi-mahi topped with mango salsa.

27. Mild Beef Stew

Prep time: 15 mins

Cooking time: 45 mins

Servings: 4

Ingredients:

- One lb. lean beef, cubed
- One cup carrots, diced
- One cup potatoes, cubed
- Half cup peas
- One tbsp olive oil
- Four cups low-sodium beef broth
- One tsp dried thyme
- Salt & pepper, as required

Tips: Use lean cuts of beef to reduce fat content.

Serving size: 1 bowl

Nutritional values (per serving): Calories: 250; Fat: 8g; Carbs: 28g; Protein: 20g; Sodium: 400mg; Sugar: 3g; Cholesterol: 50mg; Fiber: 4g

Directions:

1. In your big pot, warm up oil on moderate temp. Add beef cubes, then cook till browned. Add carrots and potatoes, then sauté for three mins.
2. Pour in the broth, then let it simmer. Add thyme, salt, and pepper. Cover, then cook on low temp for forty-five mins till vegetables are tender.
3. Stir in peas during the last five mins of cooking.

28. Black Bean Quinoa-Stuffed Bell Peppers

Prep time: 15 mins

Cooking time: 30 mins

Servings: 4

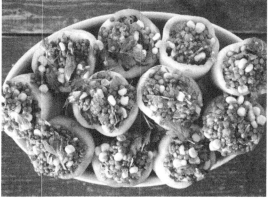

Ingredients:

- Four bell peppers, tops removed and seeds cleaned
- One cup cooked quinoa
- Half cup tomatoes, diced
- Half cup black beans, rinsed
- One tbsp olive oil
- One tsp cumin
- Salt & pepper, as required

Tips: You can add chopped spinach for extra nutrients.

Serving size: 1 stuffed pepper

Nutritional values (per serving): Calories: 220; Fat: 5g; Carbs: 36g; Protein: 7g; Sodium: 300mg; Sugar: 6g; Cholesterol: 0mg; Fiber: 8g

Directions:

1. Warm up your oven to 375°F (190°C).
2. In your container, mix quinoa, tomatoes, black beans, oil, cumin, salt, and pepper. Stuff each bell pepper with it.
3. Put stuffed peppers in your baking dish, then cover with foil. Bake for thirty mins till peppers are tender.

29. Broiled Lemon Herb Shrimp

 Prep time: 10 mins

 Cooking time: 5 mins

 Servings: 4

Ingredients:

- One lb. large shrimp, peeled and deveined
- Two tbsp olive oil
- Two tbsp lemon juice
- One tsp oregano, dried
- One tsp basil, dried
- One clove garlic, minced
- Salt & pepper, as required

Tips: Serve with steamed vegetables or over rice. Adjust seasoning to taste.

Serving size: 1/4 lb.

Nutritional values (per serving): Calories: 216; Fat: 9g; Carbs: 3g; Protein: 25g; Sodium: 300mg; Sugar: 0g; Cholesterol: 170mg; Fiber: 0g

Directions:

1. Warm up your broiler. In your container, mix oil, juice, oregano, basil, garlic, salt, and pepper.
2. Add shrimp, then toss to coat evenly. Arrange shrimp on your broiling pan.
3. Broil for three to four mins on each side or till shrimp are opaque.

30. Soft-Baked Tilapia Fillets

 Prep time: 10 mins

 Cooking time: 15 mins

 Servings: 4

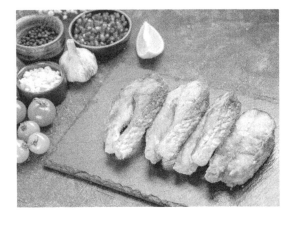

Ingredients:

- Four tilapia fillets (each about six oz.)
- Two tbsp olive oil
- Two tbsp lemon juice
- One tsp dried thyme
- One clove garlic, minced
- Salt & pepper, as required

Tips: Pair with roasted vegetables or quinoa for a balanced meal.

Serving size: 1 fillet

Nutritional values (per serving): Calories: 140; Fat: 11g; Carbs: 2g; Protein: 32g; Sodium: 300mg; Sugar: 0g; Cholesterol: 75mg; Fiber: 0g

Directions:

1. Warm up your oven to 375°F (190°C).
2. In your small container, mix oil, juice, thyme, garlic, salt, and pepper. Put tilapia fillets in your baking dish, then drizzle seasoning mixture.
3. Bake for twelve to fifteen mins till fish flakes easily.

Snacks And Small Bites

31. Mixed Berry Chia Smoothie Bowl

 Prep time: 10 mins

 Cooking time: N/A

 Servings: 2

Ingredients:

- One cup mixed berries
- One banana
- Half cup plain Greek yogurt
- Quarter cup almond milk
- One tbsp honey
- Two tbsp chia seeds
- One tbsp shredded coconut

Tips: Use frozen berries to achieve a thicker consistency.

Serving size: 1 bowl

Nutritional values (per serving): Calories: 235; Fat: 5g; Carbs: 41g; Protein: 8g; Sodium: 60mg; Sugar: 29g; Cholesterol: 0mg; Fiber: 10g

Directions:

1. In your blender, mix mixed berries, banana, yogurt, almond milk, and honey. Blend till smooth.
2. Pour it into your container and top with chia seeds and shredded coconut if desired.

32. Tender Mashed Cauliflower

 Prep time: 10 mins

 Cooking time: 15 mins

 Servings: 4

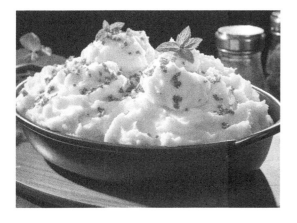

Ingredients:

- One medium head of cauliflower, chopped
- Two cups of low-sodium chicken broth
- Two tbsp unsalted butter
- One tsp powdered garlic
- Salt & pepper, as required

Tips: For extra creaminess, add one tbsp low-fat cream cheese while mashing.

Serving size: 1 cup

Nutritional values (per serving): Calories: 70; Fat: 4g; Carbs: 5g; Protein: 2g; Sodium: 60mg; Sugar: 1g; Cholesterol: 10mg; Fiber: 2g

Directions:

1. In your big pot, let broth boil. Add cauliflower, then cook for ten to fifteen mins till tender. Drain the cauliflower and transfer to your container.
2. Add the unsalted butter and powdered garlic. Mash the cauliflower till smooth and creamy. Flavor it with salt and pepper.

33. Soft Steamed Carrots and Peas

Prep time: 5 mins

Cooking time: 10 mins

Servings: 4

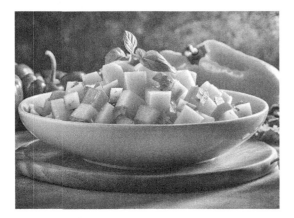

Ingredients:

- Two cups baby carrots
- Two cups frozen peas
- One tbsp olive oil
- One tsp dried dill
- Salt & pepper, as required

Tips: For added flavor, squeeze fresh lemon juice over the vegetables before serving.

Serving size: 1 cup

Nutritional values (per serving): Calories: 65; Fat: 2g; Carbs: 12g; Protein: 2g; Sodium: 20mg; Sugar: 6g; Cholesterol: 0mg; Fiber: 4g

Directions:

1. In a steamer basket, steam the baby carrots for five mins. Add the frozen peas to the steamer basket and continue steaming for an additional five mins till both vegetables are tender.
2. Transfer the steamed vegetables to your container. Drizzle with olive oil, then sprinkle with dried dill. Flavor it with salt and pepper.

34. Rice Flour Blueberry Muffins

Prep time: 10 mins

Cooking time: 20 mins

Servings: 6

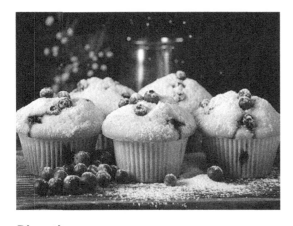

Ingredients:

- One cup rice flour
- Half cup rice milk
- One fourth cup blueberry puree
- One fourth cup honey
- One tsp baking powder
- One tsp vanilla extract

Tips: Fresh or frozen blueberries can be used.

Serving size: 1 muffin

Nutritional values (per serving): Calories: 110; Fat: 2g; Carbs: 21g; Protein: 1g; Sodium: 70mg; Sugar: 10g; Cholesterol: 0mg; Fiber: 1g

Directions:

1. Warm up your oven to 375°F (190°C). In your container, mix rice flour and baking powder.
2. In another container, mix rice milk, blueberry puree, honey, and vanilla. Combine it with rice flour mixture till blended.
3. Pour it into your muffin cups. Bake for twenty mins or till a toothpick comes out clean.

35. Mild Applesauce Cinnamon Blend

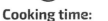

Prep time: 5 mins

Cooking time: 5 mins

Servings: 4

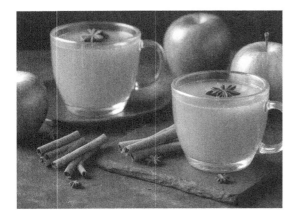

Ingredients:

- One cup unsweetened apple-sauce
- One tsp ground cinnamon
- One tbsp honey

Tips: Use organic unsweetened applesauce for the best flavor and nutritional value.

Serving size: 1/4 cup

Nutritional values (per serving): Calories: 55; Fat: 0g; Carbs: 14g; Protein: 0g; Sodium: 0mg; Sugar: 13g; Cholesterol: 0mg; Fiber: 1g

Directions:

1. In your small saucepan, warm up applesauce on moderate temp. Mix in ground cinnamon and honey.
2. Continue stirring till blended and heated through. Serve.

36. Mashed Potato and Broccoli Bites

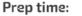

Prep time: 10 mins

Cooking time: 20 mins

Servings: 4

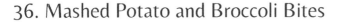
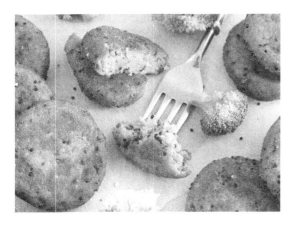

Ingredients:

- Two cups mashed potatoes
- One cup finely chopped steamed broccoli
- One-quarter cup grated cheddar cheese
- Two tbsp plain Greek yogurt
- One tsp powdered garlic
- One-quarter tsp salt
- One-quarter tsp black pepper

Tips: Ensure the broccoli is finely chopped to blend seamlessly with the potatoes.

Serving size: 4 bites

Nutritional values (per serving): Calories: 80; Fat: 3g; Carbs: 10g; Protein: 3g; Sodium: 200mg; Sugar: 1g; Cholesterol: 5mg; Fiber: 2g

Directions:

1. Warm up your oven to 375°F (190°C).
2. In your big container, mix mashed potatoes, steamed broccoli, cheddar cheese, Greek yogurt, powdered garlic, salt, and black pepper.
3. Scoop tbsp-sized portions of the mixture and shape into small bites. Put bites on your lined baking sheet. Bake for twenty mins or till golden brown.

37. Pureed Pear and Ginger Mix

Prep time: 5 mins

Cooking time: 15 mins

Servings: 2

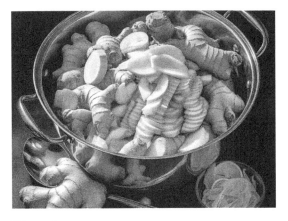

Ingredients:

- Two ripe pears, peeled and cored
- One-half inch fresh ginger root, peeled and sliced thinly
- One-half cup water

Tips: Strain the puree if you prefer a smoother consistency.

Serving size: 1/2 cup

Nutritional values (per serving): Calories: 55; Fat: 0g; Carbs: 14g; Protein: 0g; Sodium: 5mg; Sugar: 10g; Cholesterol: 0mg; Fiber: 3g

Directions:

1. In your small saucepan, mix pears, ginger slices, and water. Let it boil on moderate-high temp.
2. Cover, then simmer for fifteen mins till pears are tender. Remove, then cool slightly.
3. Transfer the mixture to your blender, then puree till smooth.

38. Soft Boiled Chicken Strips with Herbs

Prep time: 10 mins

Cooking time: 15 mins

Servings: 4

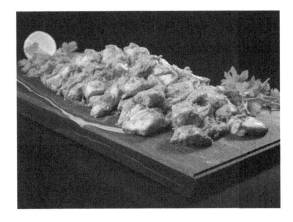

Ingredients:

- One lb. chicken breast strips
- Two cups low-sodium chicken broth
- One tbsp olive oil
- One tsp thyme, dried
- One tsp rosemary, dried
- One clove garlic, minced

Tips: Serve with steamed vegetables or mashed potatoes for a complete meal.

Serving size: 6 oz.

Nutritional values (per serving): Calories: 200; Fat: 6g; Carbs: 2g; Protein: 32g; Sodium: 200mg; Sugar: 0g; Cholesterol: 75mg; Fiber: 0g

Directions:

1. In your pot, let broth boil. Add chicken strips, then cook for ten to twelve mins till tender. Remove the chicken strips, then put aside.
2. Warm up oil in your pan on moderate temp, add garlic, thyme, and rosemary, then sauté for one minute.
3. Add the boiled chicken strips, then cook for an additional two to three mins.

1.

39. Blended Melon and Mint Cooler

Prep time: 5 mins

Cooking time: N/A

Servings: 4

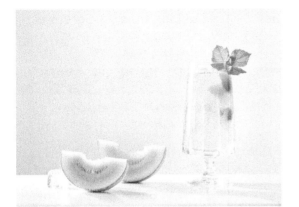

Ingredients:

- Two cups cubed cantaloupe melon
- One cup water
- Ten fresh mint leaves
- One tbsp honey (optional)
- Juice of one lime

Tips: Use cold cantaloupe for an extra refreshing drink.

Serving size: 1 cup

Nutritional values (per serving): Calories: 45; Fat: 0g; Carbs: 11g; Protein: 1g; Sodium: 10mg; Sugar: 9g; Cholesterol: 0mg; Fiber: 1g

Directions:

1. Put cantaloupe cubes, water, mint leaves, honey (if using), and lime juice into your blender.
2. Blend till smooth, then serve.

40. Mango-Banana Smoothie

Prep time: 4 mins

Cooking time: N/A

Servings: 2

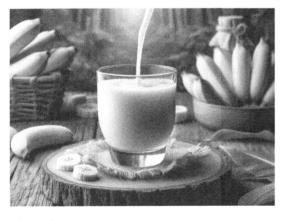

Ingredients:

- One cup of mango
- One ripe banana
- One cup almond milk
- One tbsp honey (optional)
- Half tsp vanilla extract
- Half cup of ice cubes

Tips: Use ripe fruit for a naturally sweeter smoothie.

Serving size: 1 cup

Nutritional values (per serving): Calories: 110; Fat: 1g; Carbs: 24g; Protein: 1g; Sodium: 90mg; Sugar: 19g; Cholesterol: 0mg; Fiber: 3g

Directions:

1. Put mango, banana, almond milk, honey (if using), vanilla, and ice cubes into your blender.
2. Blend till smooth, then serve.

Desserts and Treats
. . .

41. Coconut Water Jello Cubes

Prep time:	Cooking time:	Servings:
15 mins + chilling time	N/A	6

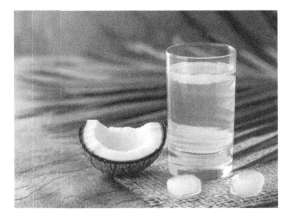

Ingredients:

- Two cups of pure coconut water
- One tbsp gelatin powder
- Two tbsp honey or maple syrup

Tips: For added flavor, you can mix in a splash of vanilla extract.

Serving size: 1 cube

Nutritional values (per serving): Calories: 25; Fat: 0g; Carbs: 6g; Protein: 1g; Sodium: 20mg; Sugar: 5g; Cholesterol: 0mg; Fiber: 0g

Directions:

1. Pour one cup of coconut water into your saucepan, then sprinkle the gelatin powder over it. Let it sit for two mins.
2. Heat the saucepan on low, stirring constantly till the gelatin is fully dissolved. Remove, then mix in the remaining coconut water and honey.
3. Pour it into your square baking dish, then refrigerate for at least two hours, or till firm. Once set, cut into cubes and serve.

42. Pumpkin Rice Pudding

Prep time:	Cooking time:	Servings:
5 mins	30 mins	4

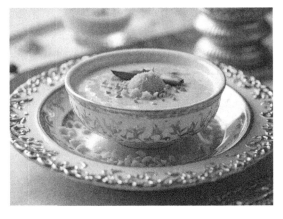

Ingredients:

- One cup white rice
- Two cups water
- One (fifteen oz.) can pumpkin puree
- Two cups almond milk
- One-half cup maple syrup
- One tsp ground cinnamon
- One-half tsp ground nutmeg

Tips: Use pure pumpkin puree without added sugars or spices.

Serving size: 1 cup

Nutritional values (per serving): Calories: 240; Fat: 3g; Carbs: 50g; Protein: 4g; Sodium: 70mg; Sugar: 15g; Cholesterol: 0mg; Fiber: 3g

Directions:

1. Cook the rice in water according to package instructions till tender.
2. In a separate pot, mix pumpkin puree, almond milk, maple syrup, cinnamon, and nutmeg. Heat on medium till warm.
3. Stir the cooked rice and cook over low heat for five to ten mins, stirring occasionally, till thickened. Let cool slightly before serving.

43. Almond Milk Ice Cream

Prep time:
10 mins + freezing time

Cooking time:
N/A

Servings:
4

Ingredients:

- Two cups almond milk
- One-half cup almond butter
- One-third cup maple syrup
- One tsp vanilla extract
- Pinch of sea salt

Tips: Add small fruit pieces or nuts for texture if desired.

Serving size: ½ cup

Nutritional values (per serving): Calories: 225; Fat: 14g; Carbs: 20g; Protein: 6g; Sodium: 90mg; Sugar: 12g; Cholesterol: 0mg; Fiber: 3g

Directions:

1. In a blender, mix milk, almond butter, maple syrup, vanilla, and sea salt. Blend till smooth.
2. Pour it into your ice cream maker and churn according to manufacturer's instructions. Transfer to a container and freeze overnight or till firm.

44. Lemon Gelatin Dessert

Prep time:
10 mins

Cooking time:
N/A

Servings:
4

Ingredients:

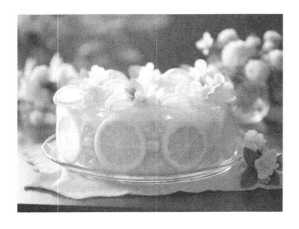

- Two cups water
- One package lemon gelatin mix (sugar-free)
- One tbsp lemon juice
- One cup cold water
- One cup ice cubes

Tips: You can garnish with a slice of lemon or a mint sprig for presentation.

Serving size: 1/2 cup

Nutritional values (per serving): Calories: 5; Fat: 0g; Carbs: 0g; Protein: 0g; Sodium: 35mg; Sugar: 0g; Cholesterol: 0mg; Fiber: 0g

Directions:

1. Boil two cups of water. Dissolve the lemon gelatin mix in the boiling water. Stir in one tbsp lemon juice.
2. Add cold water and ice cubes, then stir till the ice is melted. Pour into dessert dishes and refrigerate till firm, about thirty to forty-five mins.

2.

45. Creamy Avocado Pudding

 Prep time: 10 mins

 Cooking time: N/A

 Servings: 4

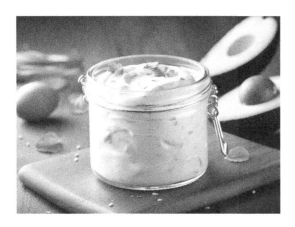

Ingredients:

- Two ripe avocados
- One-quarter cup cocoa powder (unsweetened)
- One-third cup honey
- Half tsp vanilla extract
- Half cup almond milk

Tips: For a smoother texture, ensure avocados are ripe and blend thoroughly.

Serving size: 1/4 cup

Nutritional values (per serving): Calories: 230; Fat: 15g; Carbs: 24g; Protein: 3g; Sodium: 74mg; Sugar: 18g; Cholesterol: 0mg; Fiber: 18g

Directions:

1. In a blender, mix avocados, cocoa powder, honey or maple syrup, vanilla extract, and almond milk. Blend till smooth and creamy.
2. Spoon the pudding into serving bowls and chill in the refrigerator for at least fifteen to twenty mins before serving.

46. Coconut Macaroons

 Prep time: 15 mins

 Cooking time: 25 mins

 Servings: 12

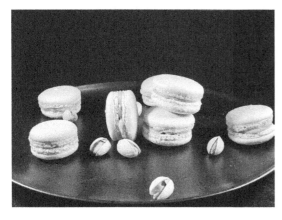

Ingredients:

- Two cups shredded coconut
- Half cup almond flour
- One-third cup maple syrup
- One tsp vanilla extract
- Two large egg whites

Tips: Store in an airtight container for up to three days.

Serving size: 1 macaroon

Nutritional values (per serving): Calories: 85; Fat: 6g; Carbs: 8g; Protein: 2g; Sodium: 30mg; Sugar: 4g; Cholesterol: 0mg; Fiber: 2g

Directions:

1. Warm up your oven to 350°F (177°C). In your big container, mix shredded coconut, almond flour, maple syrup, vanilla extract, and egg whites.
2. Scoop tbsp-sized mounds onto your lined baking sheet. Bake for twenty to twenty-five mins or till golden brown. Cool on a wire rack before serving.

47. Raspberry Oat Bars

Prep time: 20 mins   **Cooking time:** 40 mins   **Servings:** 9

Ingredients:

- One & half cups rolled oats
- Half cup almond flour
- Quarter cup coconut oil, melted
- One-third cup maple syrup
- One tsp vanilla extract
- One cup fresh raspberries, mashed

Tips: Store in an airtight container in the refrigerator for up to five days.

Serving size: 1 bar

Nutritional values (per serving): Calories: 210; Fat: 11g; Carbs: 26g; Protein: 4g; Sodium: 10mg; Sugar: 8g; Cholesterol: 0mg; Fiber: 3g

Directions:

1. Warm up your oven to 350°F (177°C). In your container, mix rolled oats, almond flour, coconut oil, maple syrup, and vanilla.
2. Press two-thirds of the oat mixture into your parchment-lined baking dish. Spread mashed raspberries evenly over the crust.
3. Sprinkle remaining oat mixture on raspberry layer. Bake for thirty to forty mins or till top is golden brown. Cool completely before cutting into bars.

48. Strawberry Banana Sorbet

Prep time: 15 mins   **Cooking time:** N/A   **Servings:** 4

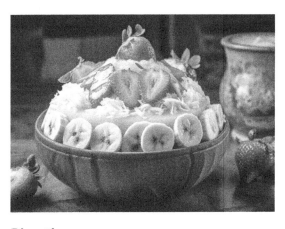

Ingredients:

- One cup fresh strawberries, hulled
- Two ripe bananas, sliced and frozen
- One tbsp lemon juice
- One tbsp honey (optional)
- One fourth cup water

Tips: Use ripe bananas for a sweeter sorbet.

Serving size: 1/2 cup

Nutritional values (per serving): Calories: 75; Fat: 0g; Carbs: 18g; Protein: 1g; Sodium: 2mg; Sugar: 15g; Cholesterol: 0mg; Fiber: 3g

Directions:

1. In a blender, mix strawberries, frozen banana slices, lemon juice, honey (if using), and water. Blend till smooth.
2. Pour mixture into your freezer-safe container, then freeze for one to two hours till firm. Scoop into bowls and serve.

49. Sweet Potato Pudding

Prep time: 10 mins   **Cooking time:** 15 mins   **Servings:** 4

Ingredients:

- One large sweet potato, peeled and cubed
- One cup coconut milk
- Two tbsp maple syrup
- One tsp vanilla extract
- Half tsp ground cinnamon

Tips: Make sure sweet potatoes are well-cooked to achieve a smooth pudding consistency.

Serving size: 1/2 cup

Nutritional values (per serving): Calories: 140; Fat: 5g; Carbs: 24g; Protein: 1g; Sodium: 30mg; Sugar: 10g; Cholesterol: 0mg; Fiber: 3g

Directions:

1. Steam or boil the sweet potato cubes for ten to fifteen mins till tender. Drain and transfer sweet potatoes to a blender.
2. Add coconut milk, maple syrup, vanilla, and ground cinnamon. Blend till smooth and creamy. Chill in the refrigerator for at least thirty mins before serving.

50. Applesauce Cupcakes

Prep time: 10 mins   **Cooking time:** 20 mins   **Servings:** 12 cupcakes

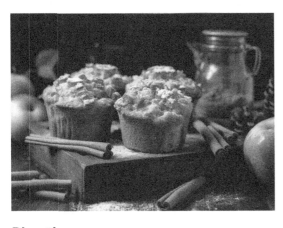

Ingredients:

- One cup unsweetened applesauce
- One cup gluten-free flour
- Half cup coconut sugar
- One tsp baking soda
- One tsp cinnamon powder
- One tsp vanilla extract
- Two tbsp coconut oil

Tips: Use a silicone muffin pan to avoid sticking.

Serving size: 1 cupcake

Nutritional values (per serving): Calories: 150; Fat: 5g; Carbs: 24g; Protein: 2g; Sodium: 90mg; Sugar: 11g; Cholesterol: 0mg; Fiber: 2g

Directions:

1. Warm up your oven to 350°F (177° C).
2. In your big container, mix applesauce, coconut sugar, vanilla extract, and coconut oil.
3. In another bowl, mix flour, baking soda, and cinnamon powder. Combine it with wet mixture till blended. Pour the batter into cupcake liners in a muffin tin.
4. Bake for twenty mins or till a toothpick comes out clean. Let cool before serving.

CHAPTER 5

Managing Digestive Symptoms

Dietary Adjustments During Flare-Ups

When experiencing a flare-up, it's pretty common for certain foods to irritate the digestive tract. The goal is to avoid those foods and choose ones that are easier on your system. Here's what has worked for me during those tough times:

1. **Stick to Low-Residue Foods:** These foods are easier for your body to digest because they leave less waste in your intestines. Examples include white bread, white rice, and well-cooked vegetables without skins or seeds.

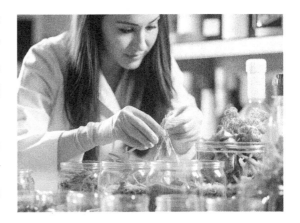

2. **Limit High-Fiber Foods:** High-fiber foods can add bulk and aggravate your symptoms. Aim for lower-fiber versions of fruits and veggies, such as bananas, melons, pumpkin, and avocados.

3. **Hydration Is Key:** Drink plenty of water to stay hydrated. Electrolyte-rich drinks can help too, especially if you're losing fluids through diarrhea.

4. **Small, Frequent Meals:** Instead of three big meals a day, go for smaller meals every few hours. It puts less strain on your system.

5. **Avoid Fats and Spices:** Fatty and spicy foods can trigger symptoms for many people with Crohn's during a flare-up. Stick to lean proteins like chicken or fish that are baked or grilled rather than fried.

Soluble vs. Insoluble Fiber

Fiber is an essential part of our diet, but it can be confusing because not all fibers are created equal. Let's break down the difference between soluble and insoluble fiber so you can make better choices:

1. **Soluble Fiber:** This kind of fiber dissolves in water to form a gel-like substance. It can help regulate your bowel movements by making your stool more solid which is something beneficial during those unpredictable times. Foods rich in soluble fiber include oats, bananas, apples (without the skin), and carrots.

2. **Insoluble Fiber:** This type doesn't dissolve in water. It adds bulk to your stool and helps keep things moving through your digestive system more quickly. While this sounds like a great thing generally, during a Crohn's flare-up, insoluble fiber can aggravate symptoms like diarrhea and abdominal pain. Foods high in insoluble fiber include whole grains, nuts, seeds, and raw vegetables.

So, what should you focus on? It's all about balance. On good days when you're not experiencing symptoms, incorporating both types of fibers is beneficial for overall digestive health.

TYPE OF FIBER	CHARACTERISTICS	SAFE SOURCES DURING FLARE-UPS
Soluble Fiber	Dissolves in water	Oats, Apples (peeled), Carrots
Insoluble Fiber	Does not dissolve in water	Whole grains (limit), Raw veggies

Probiotics and Prebiotics

Probiotics are the good bacteria that live in our gut and help keep it healthy. You might be asking yourself, *"How do I get these good bacteria?"* Well, they come from certain foods and supplements. Yogurt is one of the most well-known sources of probiotics. Look for yogurt that says "live and active cultures" on the label. Kefir, kimchi, sauerkraut, and some types of pickles are also great.

On the flip side, we have prebiotics. **Prebiotics** are like food for the probiotics; they help them grow and thrive in your gut. Foods rich in prebiotics include garlic, onions, bananas, and whole grains. Combining both probiotics and prebiotics can help create a healthier balance in your gut microbiome.

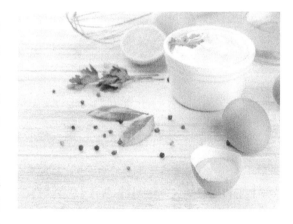

A simple example meal could be a yogurt parfait made with Greek yogurt (probiotic), topped with sliced bananas (prebiotic) and a sprinkle of granola made from whole grains (prebiotic). Incorporating these foods gradually into your diet can really help with managing symptoms.

Stress Reduction Techniques

Now let's touch on stress reduction techniques because yes, stress has a huge impact on our digestion too! Physical exercise can work wonders—simple activities like walking or stretching can help calm your mind. Meditation and deep-breathing exercises are great too. Just taking five minutes to focus on your breathing can help you feel more at ease. Mindfulness meditation is about staying present in the moment; this can reduce stress significantly over time.

Another thing to look into is yoga. Not only does it stretch out your muscles and strengthen your body, but it's also incredibly soothing for the mind. Finally, don't underestimate the power of hobbies or activities that you enjoy. Whether it's painting, gardening, or reading a good book—spending time on things that make you happy is crucial.

TECHNIQUE	EXAMPLE ACTIVITIES
Physical Exercise	Walking, stretching
Meditation	Deep-breathing exercises
Yoga	Various poses focusing on mindfulness
Hobbies	Painting, gardening

When to Consult a Healthcare Professional

Sometimes despite all our best efforts with diet and stress management, we still need medical advice. It's essential to know when it's time to consult a healthcare professional. If you notice any drastic changes in your symptoms or if they become unmanageable despite sticking to dietary adjustments and stress-reduction techniques—reach out for help. Severe pain, persistent diarrhea or constipation, weight loss that you can't explain—these are all signs you should not ignore.

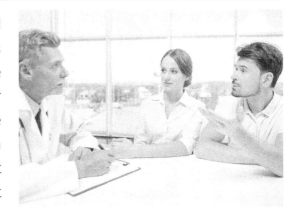

It's always better to be proactive rather than waiting until things get worse. Keeping an open line of communication with your healthcare provider ensures you're not alone in managing this disease. They may suggest new treatments or tests to better understand what's going on inside you.

Conclusion

· · ·

Coming to the end of *"The Crohn's Disease Cookbook: The Ultimate Guide to Digestive Health,"* I feel like we've covered a lot of ground together. If you've been living with Crohn's or supporting someone who is, you know how critical it is to find ways to manage this condition effectively. This cookbook provided not just recipes but a deeper understanding of how food affects our digestive health.

One of the most important takeaways from the book is how much diet plays a role in managing Crohn's disease. It's clear that what we eat can directly impact how we feel. We've learned that certain foods can trigger flare-ups, while others can support digestion and reduce symptoms. This book aimed to empower you with the knowledge and tools needed to make informed choices about your diet.

The 28-day meal plan was designed as a practical guide to get you started on a path towards better health. By laying out daily meal ideas and aligning them with nutritional goals, this plan helps take away some of the guesswork associated with meal planning. The recipes are not only tailored to be gentle on the digestive system but also ensure that you're getting essential nutrients, which are sometimes hard to absorb with Crohn's.

Speaking of recipes, there's a broad variety of options—from breakfasts and lunches to dinners and snacks. They've kept in mind the importance of flexibility, knowing that everyone's experience with Crohn's is different. Some days might require simpler, more soothing meals if you're experiencing a flare-up. That's why tips for adjusting the meal plan were included, so you can modify your diet based on your current condition.

Another significant aspect of managing Crohn's is understanding the roles of soluble and insoluble fibers in your diet. Soluble fiber can help manage diarrhea by absorbing excess water whereas insoluble fiber adds bulk to stools, aiding regular bowel movements. Learning these differences allows you to tailor your diet more closely to your needs.

Probiotics and prebiotics were also highlighted as crucial elements for maintaining gut health. They help maintain a healthy balance of gut bacteria, which is vital for digestion and overall well-being. Incorporating them into your diet through food or supplements can be beneficial.

Stress management techniques were touched upon because stress has been shown to exacerbate Crohn's symptoms in many people. Simple practices such as mindfulness, meditation, or even just ensuring adequate rest can make a significant difference in how you feel day-to-day.

Finally, it's important to remember that while dietary changes can be incredibly beneficial, they should complement other treatments and regular consultations with your healthcare professional. Each person's experience with Crohn's is unique, so working closely with healthcare providers ensures you're getting comprehensive care.

This book aimed to be more than just a collection of recipes; it's a resource offering insights into how diet impacts Crohn's disease and provides practical solutions for better management of the condition. It's about taking small steps every day towards digestive empowerment and overall well-being.

APPENDICES: Additional Resources

Supplement Guide

Navigating the world of supplements can be overwhelming, but I've put together a list of common supplements that people with Crohn's sometimes find helpful. Remember, it's crucial to consult with your healthcare provider before adding any new supplement to your routine—they can help ensure it won't interfere with your current medications or treatments.

1. **Probiotics**: Probiotics are beneficial bacteria that can help maintain a healthy balance in your gut. Some studies suggest they can support digestive health and potentially reduce symptoms of Crohn's disease. They come in various forms like capsules, powders, and even probiotic-rich foods such as yogurt and kefir.

2. **Omega-3 Fatty Acids**: Omega-3s, commonly found in fish oil supplements, are known for their anti-inflammatory properties. These could be helpful in managing the inflammation associated with Crohn's disease.

3. **Vitamin D**: Many people with Crohn's have low levels of Vitamin D due to malabsorption issues or limited sun exposure. Vitamin D is essential for bone health and immune function.

4. **Iron**: Iron deficiency anemia is common in Crohn's patients due to internal bleeding or poor absorption of nutrients. Iron supplements can help combat this, but they should always be taken under medical supervision to avoid complications.

5. **Calcium**: Crohn's disease can interfere with calcium absorption which is crucial for bone strength. Calcium supplements might be necessary, especially if you are taking steroids which can weaken bones over time.

SUPPLEMENT	POTENTIAL BENEFIT	COMMON FORM
Probiotics	Gut health	Capsules, powders
Omega-3 Fatty Acids	Anti-inflammatory	Fish oil capsules
Vitamin D	Bone/immune health	Tablets, drops
Iron	Combat anemia	Tablets, liquids
Calcium	Bone strength	Capsules, tablets

Eating Out With Crohn's

Eating out should be an enjoyable experience, but I understand how tricky it can be when you have Crohn's disease. Here are some practical tips to help ensure you can still enjoy dining out without worry:

1. **Know the Menu in Advance**: Before heading to a restaurant, check their menu online if possible. Many places now include dietary information or even specific menus for dietary needs.

2. **Communicate Clearly**: Don't hesitate to let your server know about your specific dietary requirements or restrictions due to Crohn's disease. Most restaurants are willing to accommodate special requests like gluten-free options or cooking methods that suit your needs.

3. **Choose Simple Dishes**: Opt for dishes that are plain and simply prepared—grilled chicken without heavy sauces, steamed vegetables rather than fried ones, etc.

4. **Request Modifications**: Feel free to ask for modifications such as having sauces on the side or substituting items like baked potatoes instead of fries.

5. **Be Cautious with Portions**: Sometimes smaller meals are easier on the digestive system, so consider sharing dishes or asking for half portions where possible.

6. **Emergency Kit:** Keep an emergency kit handy with any medications you might need and a probiotic snack like a small package of yogurt.

Maintaining A Food Diary

One of the best ways to take control of your diet is by keeping a food diary. Yes, it involves writing down everything you eat, but don't worry—it's not as daunting as it sounds. Think of it as a friend who helps you track what you eat and how it affects you. Why keep a food diary?

1. **Identify Triggers:** By noting down everything you consume and any symptoms that follow, you'll start to see patterns. Maybe you'll notice that spicy food or dairy causes flare-ups.

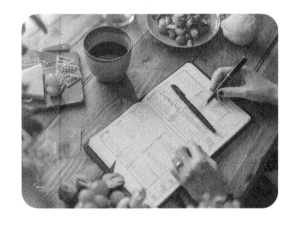

2. **Monitor Nutrient Intake:** Often, when we modify our diets, we may miss out on essential nutrients. A food diary helps ensure that you're getting balanced nutrition.

3. **Communicate with Healthcare Providers:** Your

doctor or dietitian will appreciate having this detailed information to better advise you on managing your diet.

Keeping A Food Diary Doesn't Need To Be Complicated:

1. **Start Simple:** Write down everything you eat and drink, along with the times you consumed them.

2. **Note Symptoms:** If you experience any symptoms after eating, jot those down too—be as specific as possible.

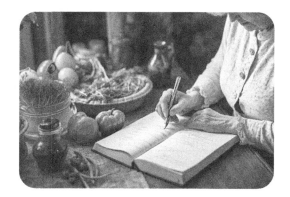

3. **Track Moods and Energy Levels:** Sometimes, Crohn's disease can affect more than just digestion. Noting mood swings or energy levels can provide deeper insights.

TIME	FOOD/DRINK CONSUMED	SYMPTOMS EXPERIENCED	MOOD/ENERGY LEVEL
8:00 AM	Oatmeal with almond milk	None	Good
12:30 PM	Grilled chicken salad	Stomach cramps	Tired
3:00 PM	Apple	None	Normal
6:30 PM	Spaghetti with marinara sauce	Bloating	Irritable

Over time, your diary will reveal how different foods make you feel, helping you make smarter choices.

Measurements And Conversions

VOLUME EQUIVALENTS (LIQUID)		
US STANDARD	**US OUNCES**	**METRIC (APPROX.)**
1 tsp	1/6 oz	5 ml
1 tbsp	1/2 oz	15 ml
1 fluid ounce	1 oz	30 ml
One cup	8 oz	240 ml
1 pint	16 oz	475 ml
1 quart	32 oz	950 ml
1 gallon	128 oz	3.8 L

VOLUME EQUIVALENTS (DRY)		WEIGHT EQUIVALENTS	
US STANDARD	**METRIC (APPROX.)**	**US STANDARD**	**METRIC (APPROX.)**
1/4 tsp	1.25 ml	1 ounce	28 g
1/2 tsp	2.5 ml	4 ounces	113 g
1 tsp	5 ml	8 ounces	225 g
Quarter cup	60 ml	12 ounces	340 g
1/3 cup	80 ml	One pound (16oz)	455 g
Half cup	120 ml		
One cup	240 ml		

OVEN TEMPERATURES	
FAHRENHEIT	**CELSIUS (APPROX.)**
200° F	93° C
225° F	107° C
250° F	121° C
275° F	135° C
300° F	149° C

OVEN TEMPERATURES	
325° F	163° C
350° F	177° C
375°F	191° C
400°F	204° C
425°F	218°C

Note: The values in the tables are approximate and should be used for reference as a guide when cooking.

Made in the USA
Las Vegas, NV
12 September 2024